P9-BYO-952

Table of Contents

There is no need to live in pain.

Getting out of pain involves changing the way you move.

Changing the way you move isn't all that hard if you are willing to focus on it for the next seventy 70 days and remain conscious of the way you walk and stand. Doing the exercises in this book that will assist you in changing the ways your body works and feels. Building muscle tone to support your posture is essential to getting out of chronic pain.

It is our belief that if you know how your body works it will be easy to make the changes necessary to help yourself out of back pain. But no one will heal you but yourself. That is the most important thing to take away from this program. Every doctor, therapist, and body worker you go to have your best interest at heart but their work will only go so far if you don't take responsibility for your own healing. The Core Walking program provides the tools and guidance that will help you change the way you walk and stand so that you can live a full life free of pain and discomfort.

3 Rules Of Thumb

1 The Body Is A Machine

Just like a car your body is designed to work in a specific fashion. Nothing in the body works in isolation—every part has an explicit function meant to work in harmony with other parts. Our skeleton is like the chassis of a car and the quality of our posture determines whether all of the moveable parts can work effectively. Many of the body's muscles though far away from each other are meant to work in synch and require proper posture to do so. Our body follows a mechanical model—it is a series of arches, hinges and pulleys, and learning about and understanding your body's mechanics will allow you to effectively utilize the genius behind the body's design.

2 Operating Instructions

You have to learn how the body works in order to use it correctly. A question I am often asked is—don't we just know how to walk? There are so many things we teach babies and young children— how to eat with a fork and spoon, how to tie your shoes and zip a jacket, but when it comes to walking, we all take our first step somewhere between ten and eighteen months old, get a big clap and a cheer from our parents and are then left to our own devices.

The fact is we are designed to walk in a specific way. Bones hold us up; muscles move us; nerves tell the muscles to move the bones. The foot is meant to fall very near to parallel with a distance of two or so inches between each foot. Our arms are meant to move in opposition to the legs with each step—when the left leg moves forward the right arm should move the same distance at the same pace. Our head is meant to be level so that the eyes can best communicate with the spine.

3 Batteries Not Included

Some people are born strong. Look at your ancestry. Where did you come from? If your forefathers were from eastern European peasantry, like mine, you likely have a reserve of strength stored away in your DNA. Our level of childhood activity goes a long way to determining the strength you carry into adulthood as well. An active child who played a lot of sports or just ran around a great deal will have a lot more core strength and body awareness than someone who spent more time indoors and avoided the playing field. There are many mitigating factors to movement as well, including illnesses, accidents, and traumas both physical and emotional.

Core Power is a very popular cultural buzz phrase. My approach to the core is about creating strength to support the muscles and bones of walking. Without the proper tone in the muscles of the pelvis and trunk, the body is not free to move effectively.

Our society's aesthetic focus is on the surface and the extremities. When most people go to the gym they work the muscles that people can see—they

What you need

Yoga Mat

Two Yoga Blocks

Belt

Tennis Ball

Timer

build strength in the arms legs and the surface of the belly. While tone in these muscle might look good, if it is pursued at the expense of the muscles responsible for holding us up and moving us we will run into trouble in the long run. The muscles of the inner thigh, the pelvic floor and deep low belly are the key core muscles for the FitzGordon Method. These three groups of muscles tend to be weak due to imbalances with their opposite more external counterparts.

Getting out of pain takes conscious effort and perseverance. Ideally you will start with the core four and move from there as you are able. But if you are in a lot of pain you might best be served by doing constructive rest for a while before engaging in more vigorous work. The core four exercises that begin the program are all very basic poses that are meant to help you isolate key muscle groups.

How To Use This Book

Another question that could be asked is when to use this book? Every body is different and each individual requires a different protocol to best access change and healing. To that end some people need to spend a lot more time on release work before getting too involved with strengthening.

You might choose to stay with the Core Four exercises of the first lesson, and other releases, for longer than the two weeks mentioned in this book. You can extend that first two weeks for as long as you feel comfortable and get to the business of deeper strengthening when you are ready for it. Honor your personal path.

I often begin the exercise portion of the program by telling clients that while I work with somewhere around one hundred exercises, you hope to need four. I can't ever overstate the role of balanced core tone when it comes to pain relief. Core Walking is about providing muscular support to correct movement patterns.

When you begin to do the exercises suggested in the workbook pay attention to the difficulty or ease with which you are able to accomplish the given task. You will notice the numbers 1 through 5 under each exercise. The first time you do an exercise grade the level of difficulty with 5 being the most difficult. Over time a 5 wants to become a 1. Once it does you can move on to a maintenance practice doing that exercise once a week or more if you would like. We are trying to build a balanced body so we want to build strength where we need it and not spend time working where we don't.

At the end of each lesson there is a section for journaling. Doing the movement and postural work in the program will bring permanent physical and mental change. Journaling can take the work to an even deeper emotional level. We've provided questions to encourage you to explore what it means to change your body and how these changes can affect your life long term. Take your time with each question. We recommend that you write without stopping for at least 5-10 minutes for each question—even if it means you write the same word over and over until something comes to you. Have fun with it and see what comes up!

Explore the sensations your body feels as you begin to change the way you walk and stand. Take note of the ease and difficulty of the exercises that you are trying out. A muscle is working successfully when you don't feel it anymore when it engages. This means that it is doing its job. Use the journaling section to monitor to progress of your muscles from weak to sore to fully functioning.

This exercise book offers one release for each lesson but if you are in pain there are more releases available on our blog @ www.corewalking.com and in the books you received on the psoas and piriformis syndrome. Pain relief often requires a different protocol to get out of pain before you can begin the work of building your core and stabilizing the body in a way that will keep you pain free. This is a science project and you are your own test patient. Be conscious of the choices you make and why you are making them as you build a new you.

6

Standing Cues

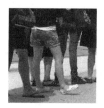

Release your butt

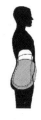

Let the belly initiate the breath

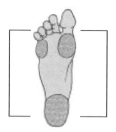

Ground evenly through all four corners of your feet

Muscles That Support The Psoas -The Holy Trinity

Our bones hold us up, and our muscles move us. I am always trying to simplify and reduce things to easily understood sound bites. But it is often more complicated. In this section, we are going to look at three muscle groups, the holy trinity, that work to support the ideal positioning of the psoas. For the psoas to be the wonder muscle that it is designed to be, it must be properly situated at its top and bottom, and it can't find that placement by itself. These groups are the adductors, muscles of the inner thigh; the levator ani, muscles of the pelvic floor; and the eight abdominal muscles.

The Inner Thighs

The adductors, the inner-thigh muscles, move the leg in toward the midline,

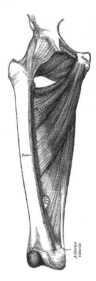

and they help stabilize the pelvis. There are five of them. The shortest of them is the pectinius, which attaches high up on the inner thigh and into the pelvis. The gracilis attaches to the pelvis and all the way down to the shin. And the three middle ones are adductor magnus, longus and brevis. All of these muscles attach around the pubic bone. But the adductor magnus, the biggest of them, has one head that attaches to one of your sit bones, the ischeal tuboroscity. Interestingly, that makes this muscle responsible for not just moving your leg to the midline but also assists with internal rotation. And that ability to rotate the leg in is an absolute key to stabilizing and setting the psoas. Proper tone of the adductors allows for the psoas to live in the back plane of the body, which, as we've seen already, is vital to good posture.

Muscle Balance

Let's take a moment to look at the concept of muscle balance. Every group of muscles has an opposite that it works with to provide stability, support and efficient movement. The opposite of the inner thighs are the outer thighs, the abductors. In all areas of the body, these muscle pairs are meant to be balanced, working in concert with all the other muscles around them to provide equal or reciprocal energy for proper use.

There are classic imbalances resulting from poor posture due to the unsuccessful employment of the psoas. In the neck, one of the most common misalignments—the ears living forward of the shoulders—creates a strong imbalance between muscles on the front and back of the neck. Most people tend to be closed in the front of their upper chest, so those muscles are short and tight and the back muscles are long and weak. It starts at the base of the body—if the shinbones and calves settle backward, the thighs are forced forward, drawing the pelvis down and causing the lower back to shorten (no pulley). As a result, the upper back falls backward and the upper chest rounds in, taking the head and neck with it.

We are supposed to be evenly balanced, with the upper chest as equally wide and broad as the upper back. Our inner and outer thighs have their own reasons why they are rarely a happy couple. One of them returns us to early childhood. Just as sitting up and crawling awaken the psoas, these movements also are a significant vehicle for inner-thigh development.

Crawling employs a dynamic stretching of the psoas and optimal use of the young adductor muscles. If employed over a length of time, when a baby pulls him- or herself up to stand, there will be beautiful balance and tone between the inner and outer thigh. To this end, it is not in a baby's interest to walk early. In fact, barring neurological problems, the longer a baby crawls the better, allowing time for the growth of core coordination. But crawling is only one issue.

Postural Imbalance

Very few of us are aligned to allow for balance between the inner and outer thighs. If you tend to stand and walk with your feet turned out, which I'd say is a large part of the population, your inner thigh would by necessity be weaker than the outer thigh—due to the position of the foot and pelvis, the inner leg turns out and is no longer in a position to work effectively.

Many of us stand this way because our parents stood this way, and so much of our learning is by imitation. Unfortunately, generation after generation of bad posture will haunt us until we get it right. Think about your parents and siblings and try to figure out whose posture and body type you inherited, if one more than the other. Figure out who you move and walk like and then try to decipher why that might be the case. It might not be a parent. It could be an older sibling that you bonded with or an aunt whom you loved dearly. That which we become is a tapestry of so many threads.

So what does this imbalance bring us? Outer-thigh dominance tends to pull us toward external rotation, which really complicates things. Your deep gluteal muscles are designed to function as both internal and external rotators. The problem is that these designs are based on the ideal. Should you stand up straight and have both feet pointing forward and not too far apart, the gluteals would be positioned in such a way that they could serve both

Walking Cues

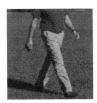

Hinge the Body to Walk

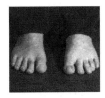

Feel the whole foot with each step

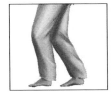

Short stride(s)

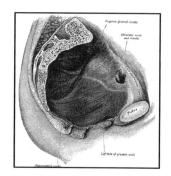

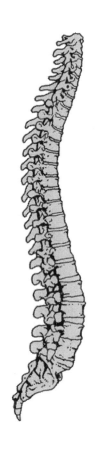

functions. Half of their span would be toward the front plane of the body, and half would be toward the back.

Try standing with the feet together, the eyes closed, and the big buttock muscle, gluteus maximus, relaxed, and see if you can sense what is going on deep inside. The gluteals are dynamically going back and forth in search of a stable place between inner and outer rotation. Now turn the feet out and move them apart. It is likely that the pelvis shuts down energetically, its joints become somewhat locked, and the inner rotation of the thighs, which is always key to the psoas, is gone.

Building proper tone in the inner thighs is imperative if we want to get our legs under our pelvis for proper posture. The psoas can't live in the back plane of the body without the help of balanced leg muscles.

The Pelvic Floor

The muscles of the pelvic floor are called the levator ani. Three muscles form a sling at the bottom of the pelvis that connects the tailbone to the pubis. This mass of muscle, about the thickness of your palm, is responsible for holding the pelvis organs in place and for control of rectal and urogenital function. Not only are these muscles bearing a lot of weight from above; they are also pierced by orifices that weaken the pelvic floor merely by their presence. Continence is high on my list of priorities, and the pelvic floor and continence are dancing partners that we must train and respect. Because these muscles are involved with your eliminative functioning, they have more resting tone than any other muscle in the body and are almost always active—or you'd be peeing all night long.

The pelvis and the muscles surrounding it serve a role unique to bipedal mammals. Just like the psoas, which is relatively dormant in quadrupeds (hence the tenderness of its loin) but wakes up when standing upright brings it into positive tension across the rim of the pelvis, the pelvic floor has a greatly different role in the biped. If you think of a dog or a cat or a horse, their pelvis is the back wall of the body rather than the floor. This leaves the organs in a dog to rest on the belly. In standing bipeds, the organs sit right on top of this muscle group, which frankly has enough to do without its newfound responsibility. Kegels exercises were created to help women with post-pregnancy incontinence issues. I think these exercises are the most important exercises any of us can do (we will learn to build the inner thighs and do kegels in the third e-book in this series).

When you have strength in the pelvic floor, what you're getting is a stable pelvis, and the stability of the pelvis allows for the psoas to move across the rim of the pelvis and have a proper, strong, toned gliding action on its journey to being a pulley.

The Abs

The last group of muscles we'll look at is the abdominals, equally important for many different reasons. You have eight abdominal muscles—four pairs. All four sets of these muscles move in different directions.

Muscles of the Trunk

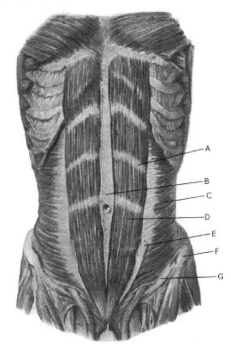

As we look at a cross section of the trunk (right), notice the way the abdominal muscles are all connected, both through the tendons and the fascia.

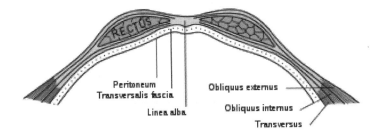

The deepest of them is the transverse abdominus. It wraps from the back to the front, meeting at the linea alba. We often refer to the transverse as one muscle, but it is two muscles that meet in the middle. This deep muscle when properly toned, provides a great deal of support to the lumbar spine.

The next layer of abdominal muscles consists of the internal and external obliques, which are angled in opposite directions. These muscles help in twisting, rotating, bending and flexing the trunk and are also active when we exhale.

The Six-Pack

The third set of abs is the rectus abdominus, the "six-pack." This pair of muscles runs vertically, connecting at the pubis at its base and the sternum and three ribs at its top. An anatomical aside about the six-pack: The body has interesting and different ways of compensating for dilemmas of length and space. The length between the pelvis and the rib cage is really too big for one long muscle to provide support. As a result we have tendinous insertions that fall between what are actually ten small muscles. So we really build ten-packs, but we only see six of them. This pack is formed when we make these individual muscles big enough so that they essentially pop out from the tendons that surround them. Muscle is designed to stretch; tendons are not.

Hard Muscle Is Bad

I have a clear image in my head of the guy on TV selling his six-minute abs program. He looks out at the camera with his six-pack jutting proud, but his shoulders are hunched over toward his pelvis as though he couldn't stand up straight if he wanted to. I always wonder if he is bent over to make his muscles pop or if that is his natural and proud posture.

I guess this might look good to some, but I'd like to take a moment to explain the nature of what happens to your muscles as you build them. Blood flows into muscles, passing through the endless number of fibers that make up an individual muscle. The way we build muscle is by creating micro tears in the muscle fibers; as they heal or repair, the body overcompensates in a way, replacing the damaged tissue and adding more, for protection against further damage. As we continue to build a muscle, the fibers need to have somewhere to go, and they begin laying down on top of one another. As more mass develops, the layering becomes denser and harder. At a certain density, blood flow will begin to become inhibited.

Just as the tight psoas results in back and other problems, a tight rectus can bring its own set of problems. Depending on the individual, breathing, digestion, circulation, and even the flow of nervous energy can be impaired.

The cultural arena of our body is a fascinating one. We have so many compensatory patterns due to the way we feel and look. We tuck our pelvis because we think our butt is too big, we hunch our shoulders to hide our breasts or because we don't like being tall. There are many more to add to this list, but I am really fascinated by the desire for six-pack abs. Our society lives in worship of the sit-up or crunch, thinking it is an express train to beauty.

Whether you think they are beautiful or not doesn't matter compared to knowing what they do and how they are connected to all of the other abdominal muscles. When we look at the cross section again it should become clear that because these muscles are connected to one another, they need to have equal tone. Imagine if one set were way stronger than the other, as tends to be the case with the rectus abdominus: As one muscle gets stronger, the other groups become weaker. We have to step back to find a new approach to balanced muscle building.

The fact that every muscle is designed to carry out a specific function has little bearing on what that muscle actually does. The brain might have a wish list in terms of a nervous response to a given stimulus, but a dominant muscle will take over ten out of ten times. With regard to the abs, it is the rectus abdominus that tends to engage at the expense of all the other abdominals.

These ß aid in breathing and help all movements of the trunk and pelvis, and for the purpose of the psoas they go a long way toward stabilizing the vertebrae and reducing stress on the spine.

Hopefully you are beginning to see that if these muscles are connected, they need to have equal tone. If they don't, and one of the four groups is stronger than the other, the other three groups are going to get weaker. The other, more pleasant scenario is that it is almost guaranteed that your psoas can find its proper place if these three muscle groups, the holy trinity of the inner thighs, pelvic floor and the abdominals, are toned and living in their proper places.

Every group of muscles has an opposite that it works with to provide stability, support and efficient movement.

The Core Four

Constructive Rest Position

Kegels

Feet Three Inches off of the Floor

Block Between the Thighs

Constructive Rest Position (CRP)

Implementation -Every morning and/or evening for 30 minutes

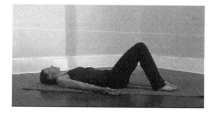

Lesson 1: Exercises

Construction Rest Position (CRP)

This is the main psoas release that we work with. It is a gravitational release of the psoas that allows the force of gravity to have its way with the contents of the trunk and the deep core.

- Lie on your back with your knees bent and your heels situated 12 to 16 inches away from your pelvis, in line with your sit bones.

- You can tie a belt around the middle of the thighs. This is a good thing to do, especially if you are weak in the inner thighs. You want to be able to really let go here and not have to think too much about the position of your legs.

- Then do nothing. You want to allow the body to let whatever happens to it come and go. Discomfort arises from conditioned muscular patterns. Try to allow the body to release rather than shift or move when unpleasant sensations arise.

- You are hoping to feel sensation that is something you can sit with and allow it to pass.

- Try to do this for 30 minutes a day, twice a day if there is a pain or injury issue—in the morning and at night. If you have time, longer sessions are advisable.

But we are not here to suffer. If sensations come up and you feel that you just have to move, feel free to move, then come back to where you were and try again. It's possible that you'll do this exercise and not feel anything; that is fine also.

Kegels

The pelvic floor is a large sling, or hammock, of muscles stretching from side to side across the floor of the pelvis. It is attached to your pubic bone in front, and to the coccyx (the tail end of the spine) in back. Make sure not to use your butt muscles in any of these exercises.

Doing these exercises correctly will help you find the correct placement of the pelvis which is key to all of the work we are trying to do.

When you tone or lift the pelvic floor the energetic quality should be a free lift up the central channel of the spine. If your pelvis is tucked under it is likely that your pubic bone will interrupt or stop the lift of the pelvic floor. Likewise, if your pelvis is rotated too far backwards you might feel that the sacrum or the back of the pelvis stops the upward flow of the pelvis floor. You know your pelvis is in the right place if the lift of the pelvic floor goes straight up the front of the spine.

There are three layers to the pelvic floor. You are trying to find the top layer, just slightly above holding in your pee (it can be very subtle)

- Tone your pelvic floor muscles, hold for a count of five. Do in sets of ten.

- Tone and lift your pelvic floor slowly, trying to stop and start as you go up, like an elevator stopping on several floors.

- If that seems easy enough try doing the opposite, lifting the pelvic floor, holding it at the top and lowering it incrementally.

- Practice quick contractions, drawing in the pelvic floor and holding for just one second before releasing the muscles. Do these in a steady manner aiming for a strong contraction each time building up to a count of fifty.

Kegels

Level of Difficulty					
Day One	1	2	3	4	5
Day Fourteen	1	2	3	4	5

Implementation Your goal is to do 200 kegels a day for the next ten years. By that point you will have done about one million kegels and you might have a strong pelvic floor

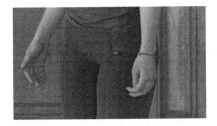

Feet 3 Inches Off the Floor

Level of Difficulty					
Day One	1	2	3	4	5
Day Fourteen	1	2	3	4	5

Implementation Begin by keeping both feet off of the ground for 5 breaths. When this is easy, and easy means no movement in the spine as well as no strain on the neck, bring the shins parallel to the floor with the knees in the original position. Hold for 5 breaths with the same criteria of ease. When this is easy extend the holding to ten breaths.

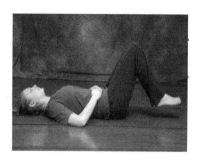

Feet 3 Inches Off the Floor

This exercise works the deep low belly muscle called the transverse abdominus. First, we're going to show how this muscle works and how another abdominal muscle, the rectus abdominus, works as well.

- Lie on your back on your mat. Bend your knees so that your feet are resting on the floor beneath your knees. Bring your hands onto the lower belly. Inhale and exhale. Inhale again and exhale but this time push the exhale at the end and see if you feel that your navel moves down to the spine and the muscle engagement is a feeling that wraps from the back to the front. Let that go.

- Now lift your head and shoulders and look at your knees. Here you should feel how when you lift the head and look at the knees, the belly pushes up into the fingers. Let the head release.

The first muscle that we engaged was called the transverse abdominis, a muscle that supports the lower back and wraps from the back to the front. The second muscle we engaged is called the rectus abdominis and connects the pelvis to the ribcage and moves in a direction straight up and down. We're going to try to isolate and engage only the deeper transverse muscle.

- Lift your right foot three inches off the floor and try to stabilize the spine as you lift the left foot three inches to meet it. Did the spine move up and the belly push up? Or did the spine actually stabilize and stay still? Release your feet.

- Starting with the second foot, lift the left foot three inches off the floor and lift the right foot three inches to meet it. Feel if the two sides were different.

- When lifting the feet without any movement in the belly or the spine becomes effortless and you can sustain it easily, bring the feet up to the height of the knees and parallel to the floor.

- When this becomes easy extend your knees forward two or three inches.

Block Between the Thighs on the Floor

- Lay on your back with the knees bent and your feet flat on the floor.

- Try to place your entire ribcage on the floor and maintain a small arch in the lower back.

- Place a block between your inner thighs between the knee and the groins.

- Engage the inner thigh muscles against the block trying to isolate them. Do your best not to use the quadriceps and outer thighs.

- Engaging the inner thighs should help you feel that your whole foot is spread evenly across the floor. Tone in the inner thighs helps you to access the inner foot.

- Don't grip your buttocks

Block Between the Thighs on the Floor

Level of Difficulty		
Day One		1 2 3 4 5
Day Fourteen		1 2 3 4 5

Implementation Squeeze the block 5X for 10 breaths. Make sure that only the inner thighs are working. Don't let the quadriceps or the outer thighs engage. Try to hold longer as you feel stronger. See if you can build up to three minutes before moving on to a more advanced version of this in lesson three.

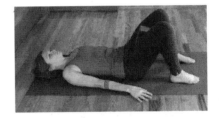

16

Write about how it feels to walk in your body. Describe any painful sensations or thoughts that come up for you.

I feel stuck and clunky when I walk. My pelvic, hips, lower back + occasionally abs and jaw are tight.

There is no flow to my movement so I do not feel good when I move.

Describe the way you walked before you began this program.
Can you identify how you learned to move a certain way? Do
you walk like one of you parents? If so, which one and why?
Have any accidents, injuries or traumas influenced the way
you move.

Write about how strong you feel in your body. How would you define strength? Are you strong?

Up until three years ago I would classify myself as strong. Since my back injury and fear of movement, I have become less fit and more weak.

What kind of exercise did you do as a child? And how did you
relate to your body back then? Describe something physical
you enjoyed as a child?

I was an active child. Swim, bike,
walked a mile to + from school

Working the core can bring up a lot of stuff. What comes up for you when you are aware of your core and working on strengthening and balancing it?

Old habits are hard to change. Are you willing to transform the way you move to get out of pain? If not, what's holding you back?

Standing Cues

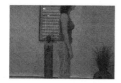

The seam of your pants are perpendicular to the floor

Walking Cues

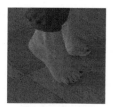

Walk on the balls of the feet

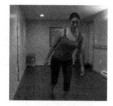

Walking is falling/ Turn the motor on

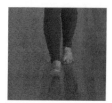

Walk to the midline

All Joints are Reciprocal

The body is a machine with a very specific design. The bones hold us upright, muscles move us, and the nerves tell the muscles to move the bones. Tendons connect muscles to the bones and ligaments connect the bones to bones. While muscles are supple and made to stretch, ligaments and tendons are much stronger and not designed to stretch much at all.

There are 206 bones in the body and they connect to each other through different types of joints that allow for different styles of movement. The knee joint connects the femur bone of the leg to the tibia of the shin. The knee is a hinge joint designed to flex and extend and nothing else. Many knee injuries occur as a result of the bones moving off their true hinge. When the knee bends the tibia and femur should stay in the same plane. There is a bit of give in the joint but we are not supposed to make use of it.

The sacrum is a gliding joint, along with the wrists and ankles. The hip and shoulder joints are ball and socket joints that allow for a wide range of motion.

All of the joints in the body are reciprocal. They are meant to work together with every movement. Take the example of walking. As you take a step forward the knee hinges up off of the ground, the hip and opposite shoulder roll in their sockets and the alternating movement of the opposite arm and leg creates a twist that involves a rotation through the lumbar spine.

Trouble arises when one joint in the chain of events doesn't work as designed. Let's look at tight hips. A tight hip refers to a limited range of motion in the aforementioned ball and socket joint that is meant to move freely.

If someone has tight hips, the knee hinges to move the leg forward but the femur that is supposed to differentiate from the hip isn't able to move successfully and the hip and the femur basically move together as one piece. The lower spine can still rotate if the arms and legs move in opposition but the rotation that should come from the hips joint will have to come from somewhere else. For example, if the ball and socket of the hip won't rotate, very often the knee is asked to twist a little to accommodate the tight hip. If the knee does hinge correctly, the lumbar spine will be asked to make up for the missing rotation in the hip. This is one of the main factors leading to lower back, hip and knee pain.

If you are familiar with yoga the transition from the pose known as chaturanga to the pose upward dog is an example of how these situations arise. As students move from plank to chaturanga they should be grounded through the inner foot with the heels parallel to each other. This alignment shouldn't change in the movement to upward dog. Instead, in many cases, students allow the heel and ankle to splay open to the side. If the ankle and foot turn open in this fashion it can't help but compromise the hip joint above it.

All joints are reciprocal and if they don't work as designed the incorrect movement in one joint will affect all of the other joints. Fluid joints are an essential component of a healthy body and walking, standing, and stretching correctly are the only ways to ensure that our body moves well.

Walking Lesson 2

- The seam of your pants are perpendicular to the floor.

- It's all about the psoas

- Walking is Falling/ turn the motor on

- Walk to the midline

Release Lesson 2: Cactus on the Back

This falls somewhere between a release and a stretch and is not nearly as benign as some of these explorations. In fact, this can be very intense, though you won't be doing much.

- Lie flat on your back. If it is not comfortable to lie with the legs straight, roll up a blanket and place it under the knees. This will release the hamstrings and reduce the strain on the lower back.

- Bring your arms out to the side and bend your elbows to form a right angle with the arms.

- Lengthen the back of the neck and allow the spine to soften toward the floor. The lower back and neck should each have a gentle arch, but ideally the rest of the spine should have contact with the floor. Move very slowly.

- Once you get your spine into a good place, bring your awareness to the forearms, wrists and hands. Try to open the hands, extending the wrists and the fingers. Move very slowly.

- Once you get the arm to a good place return to the spine. Go back and forth between the two and allow the back of the body to lengthen, soften, and release.

Cactus on the Back

Level of Difficulty					
Day One	1	2	3	4	5
Day Fourteen	1	2	3	4	5

Implementation Releasing is about relaxing into opening. Start doing this for three minutes and build up to ten minutes.

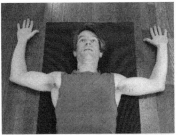

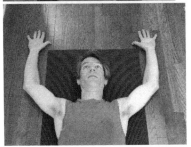

Test and Stretch Your Hamstring

Level of Difficulty					
Day One	1	2	3	4	5
Day Fourteen	1	2	3	4	5

Implementation Stretch the extended leg for 5 breaths on each side.

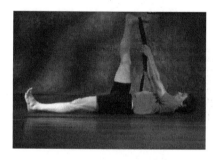

Lesson 2: Exercises

Test and Stretch Your Hamstring

Let's test the length of your hamstring. There is an ideal length and tone for every muscle. The object of our exercises is to create a balanced body. The first question is just how imbalanced are you?

We will use the hamstring muscle at the back of the thigh as our example.

- Lay flat on your back with the legs extended straight out. Have a belt handy.

- Feel how much of the body is flat to the floor. Believe it or not, everything should be flat to the floor except the lower back and the neck. This is a key component of a balanced body. Focus in on the backs of the thighs. How much space is there between the back of the thigh and the floor? The distance that the back of the thigh is off the floor is the distance that you are sinking your thighs forward when standing.

- Lift the right leg off the floor keeping it totally straight. How high can it go before the knee bends?

- Ideally with both legs straight your lifted leg should be at a ninety degree angle.

- Find the place where your leg can completely straighten. Everyone is different. Your leg might straight at a 45 degree angle to the floor instead of 90.

- The stretch itself should be in the middle of the muscle not at the back of the knee or the base of the pelvis. Depending on how tight you are, it shouldn't be hard to find a deep stretch in the middle of this muscle.

If raising your straight leg up to ninety degrees doesn't happen you should add this to your routine. Stretching tight hamstrings is fundamental to changing the position of the pelvis. Next we will offer a stretch of the hamstrings opposite muscle, the quadriceps.

Ankles and Toes

The quest for a happy body is a search for the balance of flexion and extension. This exercise offers a lot of information about your bodies imbalances. One stage is usually a lot easier than the other. They should be equally easy.

1st stage

- Point your feet bringing the heels as close together as possible. You can belt the ankles together to make it more exact.

- The idea is to get the heels to be inside of the sit bones so they can spread slightly opening the space of the pelvic floor.

- Sit up as tall as possible. Don't suffer. If this seems impossible, either come into it and out of it repeatedly or put a blanket between your calves and hamstrings to cushion the intensity.

- Spread the toes open as much as possible, trying to touch all toes to the floor. Spread tour effort evenly between the inner and outer foot.

2nd stage

- Tuck your toes under and sit up on your heels.

- Try to stretch the toes so much that the ball of the foot touches the floor.

- If it is too intense come in and out of the pose as often as needed.

If this is hard in the beginning, put a blanket under your shins and another blanket between your calves and your thighs. It is fine to ease into things over time.

Ankles and Toes

Level of Difficulty					
Day One	1	2	3	4	5
Day Fourteen	1	2	3	4	5

Implementation Try to do three sets with 10 breaths in each direction. Lean forward if you need to make this easier in order to hold for 10 breaths.

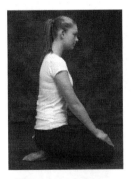

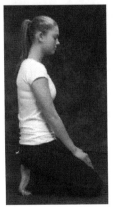

Pelican

Level of Difficulty					
Day One	1	2	3	4	5
Day Fourteen	1	2	3	4	5

Implementation Do three sets holding for 5 breaths each

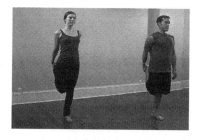

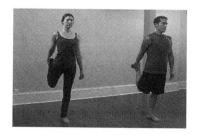

Pelican

This is a classic standing stretch that also happens to be a deep stretch of the psoas—if it is done correctly. Feel free to use the wall to support yourself.

- Bend your right leg behind you and take hold of the right foot or ankle with your right hand.

- Bring your knees in line with one another, keeping the heel in line with your sit bone. If your outer hip is very tight it won't be easy to keep the knees in line.

- Pull the right leg behind you gently. Keep the pelvis and shoulders facing forward and upright the whole time.

- Focus equally on pulling the foot back and turning the trunk forward.

- Keep the pelvic floor and the low belly strong as you try to pull the leg behind you through the balanced action of the inner and outer thigh.

If you have tight hips, it will be difficult to keep the legs aligned as you draw the right leg back. The knee will pull sideways, and it is imperative that you keep the legs in line. This is an issue with the iliotibial tract, or IT band, not the psoas, but as we know, everything is connected (no pun intended).

Core Twist (Internal and External Oblique)

This is one of our mainstay poses used to work the abdominal muscles know as the internal and external obliques. There is a lot going on in this pose. The inner thighs should stay glued together and the shoulders are resisting the urge to pull off the floor as the legs go over to the opposite side.

- Lie down on your mat on your back. Bring your arms out to the side with the wrists at the height of the shoulders, like the letter T. Turn your palms up towards the ceiling.

- Draw your knees up into your chest.

- Attempting to move the knees up, bring your knees over towards the right inner elbow.

- Looking straight up the whole time, keep the legs together and slowly come back up to the center.

- In slow motion, move the knees to the left, again drawing them up towards the elbow.

- Coming back up to the center, keep squeezing the legs together and bring the knees up towards the nose.

- To go deeper in this exercise, you're going to come over to the right again and stop about two-thirds of the way down. Stop, hold, and squeeze the legs together and release the left side of the rib cage down towards the floor. Come back up to center slowly. Move to the left on an angle as slowly as you can, stop two-thirds of the way, hover and at the same time reach the right side of the rib cage down towards the floor.

To go deeper still, the full pose is done with straight legs. The difficulty in this advanced version is keeping the legs straight, together, and moving up on an angle towards the finger tips. If the legs can't move on an angle towards the fingers you should only do this with the knees bent.

Core Twist (Internal and External Oblique)

Level of Difficulty					
Day One	1	2	3	4	5
Day Fourteen	1	2	3	4	5

Implementation Three sets three times each

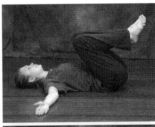

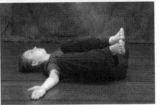

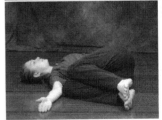

Side Stretch

Level of Difficulty					
Day One	1	2	3	4	5
Day Fourteen	1	2	3	4	5

Implementation Three sets of five breaths each

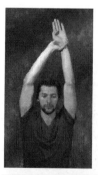

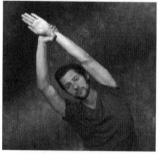

Side Stretch

The quadratus lumborum or QL is considered to be the emotional muscle in eastern disciplines. It is the next door neighbor of the psoas and responsible for any side bending of the trunk. It is one of the most important muscles for posture and movement.

- Standing tall with your butt relaxed and your thighs back under your pelvis, bring both hands over head.

- Stabilize the legs and pelvis. The pelvis should be pointing straight forward.

- Take hold of the right wrist in the left hand.

- Stretch to the left looking for the work to be between the pelvis and the rib cage.

- This is a side stretch more than a shoulder stretch.

- Pay attention to your trunk making sure that the lower back is lengthening or neutral rather than shortening.

- Soften the front ribs as you try to breathe easily into the abdomen.

Wall Stretch for Pectoralis Major and Pectoralis Minor

This is a classic stretch that is easy to find variations for (standing in a doorway with your arms on either side of the frame, and stretch forward). The muscle that stretches when the palm is turned up is pectoralis minor, one of the tighter muscles of the upper body. Everyone who feels that they are round and shouldered, almost always thinks that way because the pectoral muscles are tight. Poor posture involves both leaning backwards and rounding forwards which makes things complicated indeed.

- Stand 8-12 inches from the wall with the side of your body towards the wall. Extend your arm behind you with the palm against the wall at the height of your shoulder.

- Turn your feet and torso 45 degrees away from the wall.

- Keeping the arm well connected, stretch across the upper chest.

- Try to have the shoulders on top of the hips and ankles. The entire body would like to be equally away from the wall.

- Return to a neutral position with the torso facing forward and the side of the body facing the wall.

- Turn your palm to face up with your pinky finger against the wall at the height of your shoulder and repeat the stretch. This should be a shorter and sharper stretch of pectoralis minor.

Wall stretch for pect major and Minor/ wall stretch

Level of Difficulty					
Day One		1	2	3	4	5
Day Fourteen	1	2	3	4	5

Implementation Three sets for five breaths each

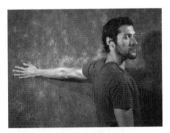

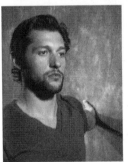

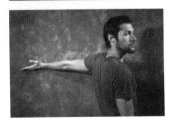

30

How are you moving differently since you began the program?
Describe the changes you're feeling, if any?

Constructive Rest Position can bring up a lot of stuff. What comes up for you when you're doing crp? Describe physical and emotional experiences, if any.

Which exercises do you enjoy or not like? Why do you think you like or don't like a particular one? Have you noticed that any of the exercises are easy or getting easier?

Besides doing the physical work, are you mentally focused on the change you are trying to bring to your body? If you are, describe how. If not, how could you bring more mental focus to this work?

You may have been struggling with pain for some time. How has your pain served you? What has it taught you?

Are you ready to let go of the pain? Is there anything keeping you holding on to it? How can you work on letting the pain go?

36

Standing Cues

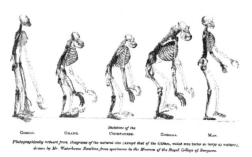

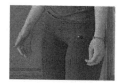

A crease in the hips

Our genus Homo sapiens sapiens – the One Who Knows He Knows – is a mere 300,000 years old, which in the grand scheme of things is not unlike a babe in the woods. This relative immaturity, combined with the fact that we are the only mammals to exclusively stand and walk on two legs, offers us something of a challenge.

Our transition to upright posture required significant adaptations of our muscles and bones. Most primates can sit and stand, with some able to walk upright for short periods of time. What allows humans to sustain these acts is the primary and secondary curves running through our whole body— most significantly those in the lumbar spine or lower back. Chimpanzees, our closest ancestors among the primates, have a flat lumbar spine and as a result can't sustain upright posture. It is our lumbar spine's lordotic or anterior curve that enables our upper body and feet to bear and transfer weight.

There are other important differences between the human skeleton and that of the chimpanzees. Our knuckle-dragging cousins use their hands to help them move forward, and although they can walk on two legs for short distances, their walk doesn't much resemble ours.

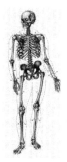

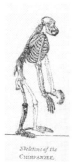

One reason for this is that our thigh bones slope inward from the hip to the knee, allowing our feet to fall directly under our center of gravity. This led us to develop powerful pelvic muscles called gluteal abductors which stabilize our bodies while in mid-stride. Chimps' thigh bones slope outwards causing them to stand and walk with their feet wide apart. What's more, their pelvic muscles are much weaker than ours, so that they have to move their entire body from side to side with each step, just to keep their center of gravity over whichever leg is bearing weight. Most importantly, chimps do not place their weight across the whole foot. Rather, they ground exclusively to the outside of the foot.

Human evolution followed many different paths. Our uprightness led to increased acuity of vision and the development of larger brains, which in turn required a wider-ranging diet including more high protein foods. To accommodate these advances, we needed to make our way down from the trees in order to forage over greater distances. In time, we began to do this exclusively on two legs.

Our descent from the treetops brought changes to the structure of our feet and the job that is required of them. The chimp foot requires an opposable "thumb" for grasping tree branches. In humans, the big toe has moved towards the midline and points in the same direction as our other toes. This seismic shift saw the big toe go from being a grasping digit to one which helps us move through space. In fact, when we are walking properly, every step ends with the entire weight of the body on the big toe.

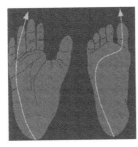

Another evolutionary change in the foot is the move towards weight bearing responsibilities and the formation of the longitudinal arch. While many primates stand largely on their toes or on the ball of the foot, human beings stand on the whole foot. The human foot is a weight-bearing platform, with spring arches that act as shock absorbers.

These transformations were necessary steps towards increased efficiency. As we evolved from quadriped to biped, our new foot became solely responsible for supporting us and moving us forward through space.

Walking Cues

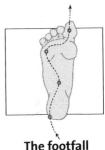

The footfall

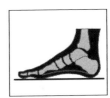

Use your arches

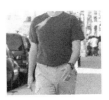

Alternate arms and legs

Frog Belly

Level of Difficulty					
Day One	1	2	3	4	5
Day Fourteen	1	2	3	4	5

Implementation Start for one minute and build up to five miutes.

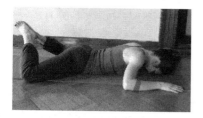

Walking Lesson 3

- A crease in the hips

- The footfall

- Use your arches

- Inner foot, outer calf, inner thigh

- Alternate arms and legs/ Rotation Through the Lumbar Curve

- The puppeteer

Release Lesson 3: Frog Belly

This is a piriformis release meant to let the piriformis shut off and stop working. But in letting the piriformis at the back relax, muscles at the front of the thigh often complain. Do your best to let it go and settle in to the sensation. But it is always important to remember that we are doing these exercises to suffer so if you need to move or come out of the pose by all means do so.

- Lay on your stomach. Bend your knees out to the side and up slightly bringing the soles of the feet together. They will likely be high off of the floor.

- The top of the pelvis and the belly should be on the floor and that will determine the height of the feet.

- Relax. Let gravity do its work on the feet. The goal is not to get the feet to the floor or anything else. It is just to be here.

- Drawing the knees higher out to the side and allowing the feet to separate slightly can deepen this a little.

- Even though this is a piriformis release you might well feel it in the hip flexor at the top of the thigh.

Exercises Lesson 3

Block Between the Thighs to Bridge

This is a return to the exercise in lesson one with an additional component that checks in with how you are using your pelvis.

- Lay on your back with the knees bent and your feet flat on the floor.

- Place a block between your inner thighs. Try to isolate the inner thigh muscles engaging them against the block them using the quadriceps, and outer thighs, as little as possible.

- Lift the hips up and continue to squeeze the block, drawing the low belly in to stabilize the spine.

- Keep your groins deep as you lift the hips.

- Don't grip your buttocks.

Did you lift your hips by tucking your pelvis under or with the natural curve of the lower back? Tucking your pelvis is old you. If you keep the curve in your lower back as you raise the hips off of the floor the spine lifts as one piece.

Block Between the Thighs to Bridge

Level of Difficulty					
Day One	1	2	3	4	5
Day Fourteen	1	2	3	4	5

Implementation Hold in bridge for one minute building up to three minutes.

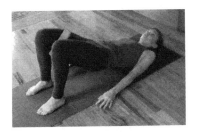

Calf Stretch

Level of Difficulty					
Day One	1	2	3	4	5
Day Fourteen	1	2	3	4	5

Implementation Start for one minute and build up to three minutes.

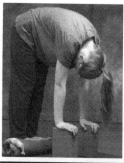

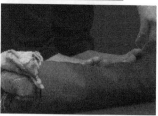

Calf Stretch

Tight calves cause more problems than most people realize. The hamstrings (which cause a lot of trouble) are essentially connected to the calves. The hamstrings attach below the knee and the calf muscles attach above the knee, and the cross paths on the way to their final destination. Very often stretching open tight calves can help to stretch the calves more successfully and sometimes bring relief to lower back pain as well.

- Roll up a blanket inside of a mat.

- Stand with your feet parallel and about two or three inches apart.

- Step your feet onto the roll keeping your heels on the floor and the balls of your feet as high up the roll as possible. Try to get as much of your inner arch as possible onto the roll

- Bend your knees softly. Keeping the center of the knees aligned over the center of the ankles, bow forward.

- Have support for your hands if necessary. (A block, or even a chair).

- Lift all ten toes if possible. Lifting your toes helps keep your arches from collapsing.

- Keeping the knees over the ankles try to bring weight to the inner foot.

Tennis Ball Under Foot

This is a gift to the body that should be with you for years to come. This is great anytime during the day. I recommend keeping a tennis ball in a shoe box under your desk; that will keep the ball from squirting away while you roll.

There is a thick pad of connective tissue on the sole of the foot called the plantar fascia. By releasing the fascia on the underside of the right foot, you effectively release the entire right side of the body.

- Place a tennis ball under your right foot.

- Spend a minute or two rolling the ball under the foot.

- You can be gentle, or you can apply more pressure. The choice is yours.

- Make sure to cover the entire foot.

Step off of the tennis ball and bend over your legs. You can check in with your body and see if you feel that the right leg seems a bit longer and looser. Feel free to scan the whole body in this fashion.

Tennis Ball Under Foot

Level of Difficulty					
Day One	1	2	3	4	5
Day Fourteen	1	2	3	4	5

Implementation Roll a tennis ball under your foot for one or more minutes on each side. Feel free to do it two or three times a day.

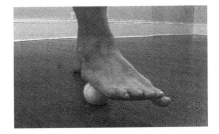

Tree

Level of Difficulty					
Day One	1	2	3	4	5
Day Fourteen	1	2	3	4	5

Implementation Start by trying to balance for thirty seconds; building up to two minutes on each side. You can add arm variations as you feel more stable in the pose.

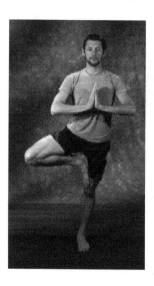

Tree

Tree pose is one of the foundations of the asana practice in yoga. I probably teach it in 90% of the classes that I teach. Balance is one of the keys to a healthy body and one of the more important factors in ageing gracefully. There are many products on the market that can help you work on your balance—tree pose is as good as any of them.

- Stand up straight with the pelvis pointing directly ahead

- Lift your right knee towards your chest.

- With the help of your left hand place your right foot high as high up the left inner thigh as possible. It is fine if the foot is not too high, just make sure not to put pressure on the knee joint if that is where your foot lands.

- Make sure your hips stay facing forward and stick your butt out so that the left leg is aligned under the hip.

- There is a tendency to lean backwards so soften the front ribs and lengthen the lower back.

- Press the foot into the thigh and the thigh into the foot.

- Repeat on the second side.

Toega

- Lift all ten toes. Spread them apart and try to place them back down with no toes touching.

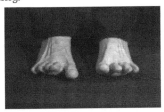

- Lift just the big toes. Place them down. Try lifting them straight up rather than towards the second toe. Even try to draw them closer to each other.

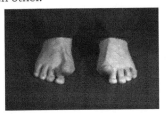 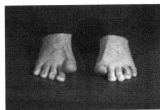

- Lift all ten toes. Place the big toes back down keeping the eight other toes up. Try to place the pinky toe down, keeping the other six toes lifted. Try placing just the fourth toes down next and so on.

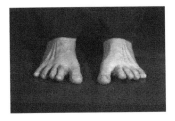 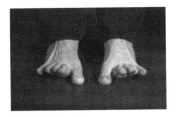

- Try lifting the pinky toes by themselves(That's me doing the best I can).

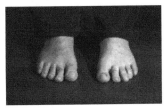

Toega

Level of Difficulty					
Day One	1	2	3	4	5
Day Fourteen	1	2	3	4	5

Implementation Have fun!

Your feet are essential to walking. How do you feel about your feet? How do you treat them? This might sound weird but, do you let other people touch your feet? Do you touch your own feet?

How does moving differently feel? Are you noticing a difference? Describe any differences.

What old you patterns have you shed so far? Which new ones have you incorporated into your daily life? Have any of the patterns been easier or harder to change? Why?

This program has both strength and release work to encourage balance. Do you relate more to release work or strength work? What appeals to you about each? What doesn't appeal to you about each?

Walking is often done without thinking about it. Now that you're focusing on the way you move, are you comfortable walking around in a new way? Do you think people are looking at you funny in New You? How can you embrace New You even if it feels awkward?

Are you comfortable doing kegels? Did you know what pelvic floor exercises were before you did this work? Can you see yourself incorporating kegels into your daily life? How?

Standing Cues

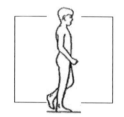

**Half the body gets a break
when walking properly**

Find Your Voice

While the psoas is my favorite muscle; my favorite bone is the hyoid. Of the 206 bones in the body, 205 of them influence the movement of at least one other bone. The hyoid bone is the only free floating bone in the whole body which means it is connected via ligaments and muscles but it doesn't articulate with any other bone.

Some anatomy geeks might make the claim that the kneecap is a floating bone but the kneecap interacts with the femur bone disqualifying it from the floating distinction. The kneecap is a sesamoid bone, a type of bone that is embedded into tendons. The presence of a bone within a tendon increases the mechanical efficiency of the muscle connected to that tendon. But the hyoid is a bone like no other.

The hyoid is the only bone of the throat— which houses the larynx, pharynx, and esophagus.
In the context of evolution the hyoid is directly related to the development of speech. There are variations of the hyoid in other animals but its unique placement in our upright posture allows it to work with the larynx and tongue to help us speak. No other animal has a larynx low enough to produce sounds and language like the human animal.

The hyoid bone is located above the thyroid cartilage and in front of the 3rd cervical vertebrae of the neck connected by a network of muscles and ligaments that sustain the hyoid bone beneath the tongue. There are nine muscles that connect the hyoid bone to the upper body. Six of these muscles are above the hyoid and three are below.

In addition to facilitating our ability to speak with the larynx and tongue the hyoid functions to support the weight of the tongue. The muscles above the hyoid are the muscles of deglutition—swallowing. These muscles form the floor of the mouth and aid in certain phases of swallowing.

These are the literal functions of the hyoid and awareness and understanding of hyoid can help us to change and improve our movement patterns.

Here are the muscles connecting the hyoid to the skeleton; The suprahyoid muscles (muscles above the hyoid), include digastric, stylohyoid, geniohyoid and the mylohyoid. These muscles connect the hyoid bone to the jaw and head. Two of the muscle below the hyoid, the sternothyroid and the thyrohyoid connect the sternum to the hyoid via the thyroid cartilage. The other two muscles that reside below the hyoid bone, the sternohyoid, and the omohyoid connect the hyoid to the sternum of the ribcage and the scapula of the shoulder girdle.

This means that the whole upper body—head, jaw, rib cage and shoulder girdle are muscularly connected through the hyoid bone and this creates interesting possibilities when it comes to movement as well as speech.

Here are two interesting hyoid facts: I take my learning anywhere I can get it, and I learned via Law and Order—the most ubiquitous show in the history of television—that as a general rule if a hyoid bone is fractured when someone suffocates, the death will be a considered a homicide. Another interesting thing to note is that the job of the omohyoid muscle that connects the hyoid to the shoulder blade is to strap down the jugular vein. As a result of this there is a small tendon in the middle of the muscle that covers the vein. If it wasn't there we would be in pain every time the jugular pulsed.

The hyoid is my favorite bone for two reasons. The first is that the vocal chords, or vocal ligaments, are situated directly above the hyoid bone running in a line from the front to the back. If the head is misaligned the hyoid is out of place. When the hyoid is out of its correct placement in the body our voice will be unable to resonate at its fullest. The opposite is true as well. If you can pull the head back into proper alignment, the voice will always be at most resonant and clear. And if your voice is at its most resonant you know that your posture has to be fairly good.
And for me the ability to get the head back where it wants to be can be facilitated by aligning the hyoid bone. When you get your hyoid to its proper place you will find your true voice. And the fact all of the structures of the upper body are literally connected to the hyoid means that an upper body that moves in harmony, moves through the hyoid bone.
One way to feel this is in the pose in yoga that is referred to as small cobra.

- Lay on your belly with the hands on the floor by your chest.

- Lift the head, neck and chest up off of the floor and try to feel what initiates the movement.

- Unfortunately we often lift from the head and the rest of the upper body follows along.

- Try doing it again, this time initiating from the hyoid bone. If you are successful the head, ribcage and shoulder girdle all move as one piece together as they come up off of the ground.

The hyoid bone and it successful use and alignment present us with amazing opportunities for postural health and function. I can't repeat enough that if you know how your body is meant to work, you are much more likely to use it correctly.

Walking Cues

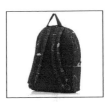

Open the middle back: back pack

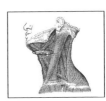

Find your voice

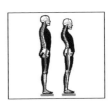

The IT band moves forward

Block Lunges

Level of Difficulty					
Day One	1	2	3	4	5
Day Fourteen	1	2	3	4	5

Implementation 2 sets for 90 seconds on each side.

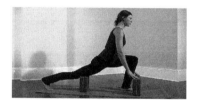

Walking Lesson Four

- Half the body gets a break when walking properly

- Open the middle back- Back pack

- Find Your Voice

- The IT band moves forward

Release Lesson Four: Block Lunges

This is a release of both the quadriceps and the psoas. Sometimes the quadriceps muscles are so tight, there is no getting to the psoas until we release the quads a bit. You'll need three blocks for this.

- Positioned on your hands and knees or in Downward Facing Dog, step the right foot forward in between your hands. Two blocks will be for your hands by the front foot.

- Place the third block underneath the quadriceps muscle just above the knee, at the base of the thigh.

- Tuck the back toes and let the weight of the body fall onto the block. Do your best to keep the heel of the back foot pointing straight up toward the ceiling.

- The front leg and hip should not be under any strain. Feel free to make adjustments, turning the foot out or stepping the foot wider.

- This is one of the few times that I will say disregard the front leg. It should be turned out and open enough that all of the feeling is in the leg on top of the block.

- You need to stay for 90 seconds to get the full benefits of this pose.

Exercises Lesson Four

Standing Pigeon

This is a deep stretch of the piriformis muscle in addition to being a good pose for developing better balance.

- Stand with the feet hip distance apart and parallel.

- Cross the right ankle over the left knee. Flex the right foot strongly (push through the heel).

- Begin to squat. Think about lowering down backwards more than leaning forward.

- Stick the butt out.

- If you can bring the forearms onto the right shin, place them there and hold. Don't worry if you can lower that far down.

- Ideally the right shin is parallel to both the front of your mat and the floor. Tight hips will cause the knee of the crossing leg to be higher than the ankle. Over time this knee should lower.

- Breath.

- Change sides.

Standing Pigeon

Level of Difficulty					
Day One	1	2	3	4	5
Day Fourteen	1	2	3	4	5

Implementation Start by trying to hold this for fifteen seconds and build up to one minute if you can.

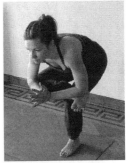

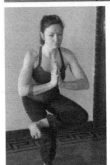

Binding and Sliding

Level of Difficulty					
Day One	1	2	3	4	5
Day Fourteen	1	2	3	4	5

Implementation Try and do ten repetitions.

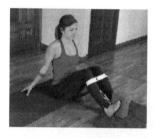

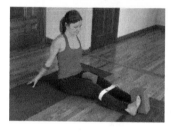

Binding and Sliding

This is a very intense position. It is an excellent exercise for tracking the legs in their correct alignment. When you are bound in this fashion the legs are forced to move straight in the way they are designed. Everything you feel in this pose is giving you information about what your legs want to do as opposed to what they should do.

- Place a block between your feet and a block between your inner thighs.

- Tighten a belt around the calves and make it as tight as you can. The belt should be a couple of inches below the knee around the meat of the calf muscle.

- Keep the big toes on the block at your feet and do your best to pull your heels slightly away from the block.

- Draw the knees towards your chest keeping your heels on the floor. Extend the legs back out.

- You don't have to pull all the way in or extend all the way out.

- Try to keep your feet even, pressing through the inner foot and drawing the outer foot back.

- The emphasis on the exercise is inner thigh, outer calf, and the mound of the big toe on the inside of the foot.

Bicycling the Legs

- Lay on your back with the legs straight out in front of you.

- Draw your right knee into your chest.

- Bring the left leg about a foot off of the floor.

- Begin to switch the position of the legs bringing the left knee in and extending the right leg out.

- Try to keep the legs in line with the hips preventing the legs from extending and pulling out to the side of the hips.

- Be aware of your inner thighs and try to use them to help initiate the extension of the leg.

- As lightly as possible rub the fabric of your pants or your bare knees together as you switch sides. You always want to move through the midline of the body.

- If this is easy focus on moving the legs at the exact same time so that they cross in the exact middle. The dominant leg wants to move much faster.

Bicycling of Legs

Level of Difficulty					
Day One	1	2	3	4	5
Day Fourteen	1	2	3	4	5

Implementation Start by trying to move the legs continuously for thirty seconds building up to one minute.

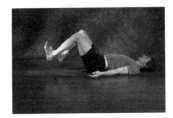

Forearm Plank

Level of Difficulty					
Day One	1	2	3	4	5
Day Fourteen	1	2	3	4	5

Implementation Fifteen seconds building to one minute.

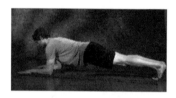

Forearm Plank

Forearm plank has been a go-to core exercise for many years. Once you have decent tone in your transverse abdominis (lesson one), forearm plank is a great way to build strength throughout the rest of the trunk.

- Lie down on your belly with your elbows under your shoulders and your palms flat to the floor in front of you.

- Lift the hips up off of the floor bringing the ankles, hips, shoulders and ears into one straight line.

- If this is difficult begin by lifting the hips with the knees still on the floor and then try to lift the pelvis up.

- Reach backwards through your heels and forward through your spine, drawing your navel up towards the ceiling.

- Be aware of the upper back. We have a tendency to round or push up the upper back and use the tightness of our chest muscles to hold us up. Try to broaden the upper chest and let the upper spine soften gently towards the floor.

Are you spending more of your time in New You or Old You? What, if anything, is keeping you from mostly living in New You? If you're mostly living in New You, describe how it feels.

Developing good posture can make your voice more powerful.
Have you noticed a change in your voice since you began?
In what ways have you been holding your voice back? How
comfortable are you expressing yourself?

Have you noticed any shift in your strength? Are you feeling stronger?

How has your pain shifted? What else can you do to continue
to move out of pain?

When you practice the exercises, do you gravitate toward the ones that you like or the ones that you need? Are you avoiding any exercises? How can you embrace the harder ones? If you're enjoying them, which ones and why?

Describe the changes you've experienced this far? How is
your body responding to the changes? How are you feeling
about the changes?

64

Standing Cues

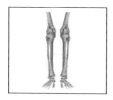

Knee tracks over the ankle

We need to think up physically, spiritually and emotionally. This is the essence of the Core Walking program. The initial focus is on the legs as we try and get rooted into the ground. But we finish trying to elevate towards the sky. The energy of the body radiates in two directions from the deep core we move down through the legs and up through the spine.

The four spinal curves move in two directions—the sacrum and thoracic spine curve out while the lumbar and cervical spine moves in. Let's look at how the spine moves. There is a great deal of movement available to the spine, though each section moves differently. The spine can flex toward the front of the body, it can extend towards the back of the body; it can stretch to either side and can pull back to the middle from that side. It can rotate or twist as well though rotation is fairly limited in the lumbar spine while the cervical spine has a great deal of rotation. It is important to note that there is not a lot of a backward bend available to the thoracic spine.

But how does the spine lengthens energetically? This is way more interesting than the simple "stand up straight" from childhood.

First, it's worth looking at why we want to lengthen the spine. Sure, it could make you taller. But there's much more going on here. Again, energetically life revolves around the spine. The Central Nervous System (CNS) includes the brain and spinal cord, which is housed inside the spinal column. The Peripheral Nervous System (PNS) connects the CNS to other parts of the body, and is composed of nerves that emanate from the spinal column. Therefore, the skeletal alignment of our spine is the key determinant of our access to the body's energetic resources. Our nervous system is the body's information gatherer, storage center and control system. Its function is to collect information about external conditions in relation to the body's internal state, to analyze this information, and to initiate the proper response. It is our energetic mothership.

To unlock this energy we must balance the curves of the spine and lengthen them in two directions; the sacrum and tailbone move down, and the lumbar spine and everything above extends up. We want to learn to lengthen the spine, while maintaining all of its natural curves in order to pull the spinal column to its maximum length. Again, this is not the throwing the shoulders back posture instruction of yore.

In order to visualize a healthy lengthening of the spine we need to understand the muscles that are involved in this action. Your pelvic floor is a group of muscles called the levator ani, the elevator of the anus. Energetically these muscles moves upward into the core of the body. Makes sense with the name. Your buttocks muscle, the big gluteus maximus, is a muscle that extends down the leg energetically flowing downward to the earth.

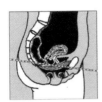 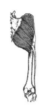

These muscles (levator ani & gluteus maximus) have specific functions that work in opposition to each other. Levator ani up. Gluteus maximus down. Unfortunately this is rarely the environment in which we live because we tend to overuse the buttocks and under use the pelvic floor and as a result the spine can begin to suffer. And as the spine suffers, we suffer. We create a compressed environment for the mothership of our nervous system.

In our experience at the walking program, we see that most people tend to overuse the buttocks. We grip in the buttocks when we're standing. Simply (and profanely put), we are a bit tight a**ed. How? If your legs are underneath your pelvis the butt can do less. However, we tend not to stand that way. Instead, we tuck the pelvis under while standing, just like when we're slouching in chairs. If the thighs begin to sink forward as they do in most people, the quadriceps (big thigh muscles) and the buttocks must work to provide stability.

Gripping the buttocks shuts down energetic movement through the spine. In standing the gluteus maximus should not be working. Repeat. When you are standing, you should not be using your buttocks. Unfortunately, our buttocks-gripping posture usually shifts the gluteus maximus into a different role of sucking energy upwards rather than down. This means that our pelvic floor weakens because it's not able to do its real job of moving energy up.

An unfortunate result of these actions is that people are working their spine from the lumbar curve up instead of from the tailbone up. I see this in yoga class all the time. You can experience this in Cat & Cow (one of the exercises at the end). If you come onto your hands and knees and begin to arch and round the spine, you can try to feel where in the spine you initiate the action. We want to move from the tail all the way to the crown but I see that most people move from the lumbar up leaving the poor sacrum and tailbone out of the action.

Walking Cues

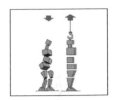

Go up - tail to crown

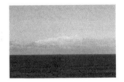

Horizon line

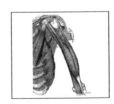

The arms hang free

Releasing the buttocks opens the possibility for one of the body's most important features: toning the pelvic floor. Toning your pelvic floor creates the upward energy that allows for the sacrum and the tailbone to move down. Now toning your pelvic floor sounds way more interesting than throwing your shoulders back right? Yet, if the idea of toning your pelvic floor doesn't make sense you can try to feel it in many ways. Holding in your pee, gently engaging between the anus and the genitals and lastly if all else falls squeeze the anus to get a sense of movement at the base of the pelvis. Ideally you will feel a shift in the bones as well as the muscles. As mentioned earlier, when you tone your pelvic floor, your tailbone should move forward ever so slightly towards the pubis or front of the pelvis as the sacrum lengthens down. Add to this a gentle tone of the abdominals and a lengthening from the back of the neck can pull the spine up into its full extension at the top.

The key aspect of this is that though the spine is moving in two directions to find its length, the muscular action is all about lifting or lengthening up. It's about lifting the pelvic floor to release the lower spine down. In the chakra system, the tailbone is referred to as the root chakra. This is where our sense of stability and connection with the world originates. When we don't stand on our legs and thrust the pelvis forward and grip the buttocks and lose the tone of the pelvic floor, we lose our connection with the root or the earth. Sure, we might be able to lift up at bit through the upper spine, but everything below the lumbar spine is diminished. In that chakra system, the energy of the body originates at the base of the tail. We can't really lift up until we have this support. Thus, we need this harmonious relationship between the buttocks releasing down and the pelvic floor lifting up. Only then can the spine lengthen in two directions and create a healthy channel for our Central and Peripheral Nervous Systems. Only by moving in two directions can we create the space to energetically thrive.

Walking Lesson Five

- Knee Tracks Over The Ankle/ The inner thigh moves backwards

- Go up- tail to crown

- The Head Floats Above the Spine- horizon

- The Arms Hang Free

- A Jaguars Engine

Release Lesson Five: Subbocciptal Muscles

The suboccipital muscles connect the base of the skull to the top of the spine and are the only muscles in the body with an energetic connection to the eyes. They tend to be chronically short.

- Lie flat on your back and bring a small natural arch to your lower back. The legs should be straight; you can put a blanket under the knees if there is any strain on the lower back.

- Raise your arms to the sky, pulling your shoulder blades away from the floor. Let the upper spine settle onto the ground as you grasp each shoulder with the opposite hand.

- Soften your grip on the shoulders but try to allow the upper spine to make contact with the floor.

- Lengthen the back of the neck as much as you can without closing off or creating discomfort at the front of the throat.

Subbpocciptal Muscles

Level of Difficulty					
Day One	1	2	3	4	5
Day Fourteen	1	2	3	4	5

Implementation If you can start by doing this for three minutes and try to increase to ten minutes.

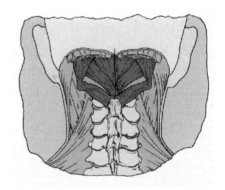

Belt Stretch

Level of Difficulty					
Day One	1	2	3	4	5
Day Fourteen	1	2	3	4	5

Implementation Do ten repetitions with the arms as wide apart as possible. Slowly bring the hands closer together as the stretch gets easier.

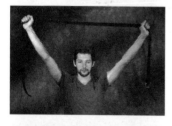

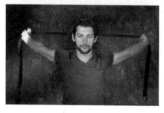

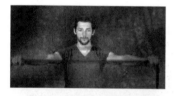

Exercises Lesson Five

Belt Stretch

This is a strong stretch of the Pectoralis minor at the front of the chest. You can even do it with a broom stick if a belt isn't handy.

- Hold a belt with your hands wide apart. Bring the belt over your head and behind you keeping the arms and wrists straight. You may need to move your hands slightly further apart for them to stay straight.

- Do your best to maintain the position of the head, neck and chest.

- There is a tendency for the head to move forward as the belt and arms move backwards. Use tone in your belly to support the head.

- Try to move both arms at the same pace.

- As this gets easier move the hands closer together.

Dying Warrior (ITB stretch)

- Starting on your hands and knees or in downward facing dog, bring the right leg across the leg side of the body.

- Do your best to bring it slowly up to the height of the pelvis.

- Stay in the position of the second picture for a few breaths before you come down to the ground. This is a stretch of the outer hip that we love more than most.

- When the hip is on the ground work on turning the top hip towards the foot on the floor. The stretch will likely move from the outer hip to the area between the pelvis and the ribcage.

- For some it will be easy to place the forearms on the floor in front of you. If not, do your best.

- Ultimately you can slip the left arm under the right shoulder bringing the left shoulder to the ground. (That is fairly advanced)

Dying Warrior (ITB Stretch)

Level of Difficulty					
Day One	1	2	3	4	5
Day Fourteen	1	2	3	4	5

Implementation Do five breaths in each phase on both sides.

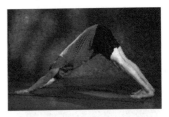

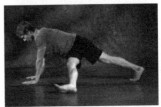

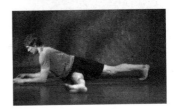

Boat

Level of Difficulty					
Day One	1	2	3	4	5
Day Fourteen	1	2	3	4	5

Implementation Do five breaths five times.

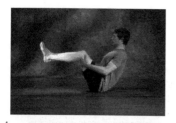

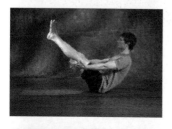

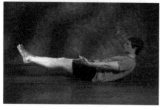

Boat

This classic yoga pose is another way to work the core and the advanced version brings the psoas in and out of engagement.

- Sit on the floor with your knees bent and the feet flat. Take hold of the back of your thighs and bring the feet up off the floor. That might be enough, or you might release the hands along side the knees.

- If possible you can straighten the legs trying to find the legs and trunk 60 degrees off of the floor. Keep the arms alongside the knees.

- As this gets easier, lean both the legs and the torso back to about 30 degrees. The back should round a bit and the work of the core should be stronger.

- Try to pull yourself back up to the original position. Repeat five times.

Inner thigh stretches (Baddha konasana/ tarasana/ Upavista konasana)

Seated forward bends are extremely difficult. The body wants to move in to distinct pieces. The upper body wants to move in a uniform way from the lower body. This means that the pelvis has to be able to rotate around the leg bones for the trunk to come forward in one piece. This is way easier said than done. If you head moves faster than the rest of your trunk in any of these variations you have gone too far.

Stage 1

- Sit with your legs straight out in front of you, raising your pelvis on a blanket if your hips or groins are tight.

- Exhale, bend your knees, pull your heels toward your pelvis, then drop your knees out to the sides and press the soles of your feet together.

- Bring your heels as close to your pelvis as you comfortably can. You can hold onto the outer feet or ankles.

- Sit so that there is a natural arch in the lumbar spine which might require sitting up one something, and might not be possible at all.

- Tone the lower belly and draw the shoulder blades onto the back and lengthen forward moving the spine in one piece towards the feet.

- Never force your knees down.

Stage 2

- Move your feet about a foot and a half forward creating a diamond shape with your legs.

- Extend forward in the same way as the first stage.

Stage 3

- Extend the legs and feet wide apart.

- Sit so that there is a natural arch in the lumbar spine which might require sitting up one something, and might not be possible at all.

- Tone the lower belly and draw the shoulder blades onto the back and lengthen forward moving the spine in one piece towards the floor in front of you.

Inner Thigh Stretches (Baddha konasana/tarasana/upavista konasana)

Level of Difficulty					
Day One	1	2	3	4	5
Day Fourteen	1	2	3	4	5

Implementation Spend five breaths each variation.

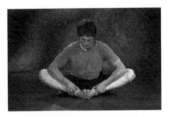

As you move better, you'll grow taller. How do you feel about taking up more space? Are you ready to accept New Taller You?

Corewalking is all about balance. Do you feel more balanced in your body? In what ways can you increase the sense of balance? How does being in balance make you feel?

74

What will you do to keep this program moving forward in your life? Can you commit to practicing the exercises that are right for you? How can you commit to living in New You?

This process is ongoing and lifelong. What is your goal for your body over the next year? The next 5 years? The next 10?

What commitment can you make to achieving your goals?
How can Corewalking continue to support these goals?

Celebrate the way you've changed your walk and changed your life. Describe Old You and New You. By saying goodbye to Old You, you make room for New You. Describe how this process went for you and recognize the hard work you've done!

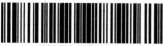

Made in the USA
Lexington, KY
12 April 2018